INSULIN RESISTANCE

COOKBOOK AND MEAL PLAN
for beginners

A diet guide to prevent pre-diabetes Lose weight and improve insulin-sensitivity with balance crafted recipes

SARAH BILLY

Table of Contents

Table of Contents....................................3

INTRODUCTION **9**

What is insulin resistance..........................9

Factors that contribute to the development of insulin resistance.........10

How Insulin Resistance Develops in the Body..12

CAUSES AND SYMPTOMS 14

Importance of Insulin Sensitivity **19**

Connection to Overall Metabolic Health 19

Role in Preventing Type 2 Diabetes.......23

Types of Insulin Resistance......................28

Common Misconceptions About Insulin Resistance..**32**

Dispelling Myths and Misunderstandings 32

Clarifying the Relationship Between Insulin and Weight Gain 37

TREATMENT AND DIAGNOSIS 43

Diagnosis of Insulin Resistance: 43

Treatment and Management of Insulin Resistance 45

28 DAY MEAL PLANS FOR INSULIN RESISTANCE DIET 50

Week 1 50

Week 2 53

Week 3 57

Week 4 61

INSULIN RESISTANCE BREAKFAST FRIENDLY RECIPE 65

Greek Yogurt Parfait: 65

Quinoa Breakfast Bowl: 66

Vegetable Omelette: 67

Chia Seed Pudding:.................................68

Blueberry Almond Smoothie: 69

Whole Grain Waffles with Berries: 70

Avocado and Smoked Salmon Toast: ..71

Cottage Cheese and Pineapple Bowl: 72

Egg Muffins with Spinach and Feta:......73

Peanut Butter Banana Smoothie:..........74

Frittata with Vegetables: 75

Turkey and Vegetable Breakfast Wrap:76

Almond Flour Pancakes:.........................77

Salmon and Cream Cheese Bagel: 78

Pumpkin Spice Overnight Oats:.............79

Egg and Spinach Breakfast Wrap 80

Cinnamon Apple Quinoa Bowl:.............80

INSULIN RESISTANCE LUNCH FRIENDLY RECIPE

....**82**

Grilled Chicken Salad with Avocado:...82

Quinoa and Black Bean Bowl: 83

Salmon and Vegetable Stir-Fry:.............. 84

Mediterranean Chickpea Salad: 85

Turkey and Quinoa Stuffed Peppers:.... 86

Chicken and Vegetable Quinoa Bowl: 88

Shrimp and Avocado Wrap: 89

Roasted Vegetable and Hummus Wrap:
.... 90

Caprese Chicken Salad:........................ 91

Tuna and Chickpea Salad:.................... 92

Spinach and Feta Stuffed Chicken Breast:
.... 93

Sweet Potato and Chickpea Buddha
Bowl:... 94

Eggplant and Tomato Lentil Salad: 95

Turkey and Vegetable Stir-Fry:.............. 96

Greek Chicken Wrap: 97

Spaghetti Squash Primavera:...................98

Cauliflower Fried Rice with Shrimp.........99

Tomato Basil Zoodle Salad with Grilled Chicken 100

INSULIN RESISTANCE DINNER FRIENDLY RECIPE...102

Baked Salmon with Lemon-Herb Quinoa: 102

Vegetarian Cauliflower and Chickpea Curry 103

Grilled Chicken and Vegetable Skewers: 104

Spaghetti Squash Shrimp Scampi:........105

Stuffed Bell Peppers with Turkey and Quinoa: 106

Baked Cod with Mediterranean Vegetables: 107

Eggplant and Tomato Lentil Casserole: 108

Grilled Tofu and Vegetable Skewers: . 109

Mushroom and Spinach Stuffed Chicken Breast: 110

Cauliflower Fried Rice with Chicken: .. 111

Sweet Potato and Chickpea Curry: ... 112

Zucchini Noodles with Pesto Shrimp: .. 113

Sesame Ginger Tofu Stir-Fry: 115

Mediterranean Quinoa Bowl with Grilled Chicken: 116

Broccoli and Cheddar Stuffed Baked Potatoes: 117

Chickpea and Spinach Coconut Curry: 119

CONCLUSION 121

CHAPTER ONE

INTRODUCTION

What is insulin resistance

Insulin resistance is a physiological condition where the cells in the body become less responsive to the effects of insulin. Insulin is a hormone produced by the pancreas that plays a crucial role in regulating blood sugar (glucose) levels. Its primary function is to facilitate the uptake of glucose by cells, allowing them to use it for energy.

In a healthy individual, when blood sugar levels rise after eating, the pancreas releases insulin into the bloodstream. Insulin then signals cells, particularly muscle, fat, and liver cells, to take up glucose from the blood. This process helps maintain balanced blood sugar levels.

However, in the case of insulin resistance, cells become less sensitive to the action of insulin. As a result, they do not respond as effectively to the hormone and glucose uptake is impaired. This leads to elevated levels of glucose in the bloodstream, a condition known as hyperglycemia.

Factors that contribute to the development of insulin resistance

Insulin resistance is a key factor in the development of type 2 diabetes. When the pancreas can no longer compensate for the reduced effectiveness of insulin, blood sugar levels continue to rise, eventually leading to diabetes.

It's important to note that insulin resistance can be managed and often reversed through lifestyle modifications such as a healthy diet, regular exercise, and maintaining a healthy weight.

Find below factors that contribute to the development of insulin resistance

1.	**Genetics:** Some individuals may have a genetic predisposition to insulin resistance.

2.	**Lifestyle Factors:** Poor diet, lack of physical activity, and obesity are significant contributors to insulin resistance.

3.	**Metabolic Syndrome:** Insulin resistance is often associated with metabolic syndrome, a cluster of conditions that includes abdominal obesity, high blood pressure, high triglyceride levels, low HDL cholesterol levels, and elevated blood sugar.

4.	**Hormonal Imbalances:** Conditions such as polycystic ovary syndrome (PCOS)

can lead to hormonal imbalances that contribute to insulin resistance.

How Insulin Resistance Develops in the Body

A key contributor is a poor diet characterized by excessive consumption of refined carbohydrates, sugars, and saturated fats. These dietary patterns contribute to weight gain and metabolic dysfunction, fostering insulin resistance. Sedentary lifestyles further exacerbate the problem, as regular physical activity is crucial for maintaining insulin sensitivity.

Obesity, especially the accumulation of visceral fat, is a central player in insulin resistance. Adipose tissue dysfunction leads to the release of inflammatory molecules, creating a chronic state of low-grade inflammation that interferes with insulin signaling. Chronic inflammation is a pivotal factor in the progression of insulin resistance.

Hormonal imbalances, such as those seen in conditions like polycystic ovary syndrome (PCOS), can disrupt insulin sensitivity. Additionally, aging introduces changes in body composition and metabolism that contribute to insulin resistance.

The intricate interplay of these factors results in a cellular environment where insulin's effectiveness diminishes. Cells, particularly those in muscle, fat, and liver tissues, become less responsive to insulin signals, leading to impaired glucose uptake. Over time, the pancreas struggles to produce enough insulin to overcome this resistance, eventually resulting in elevated blood sugar levels and an increased risk of developing type 2 diabetes. Recognizing these contributing factors is crucial for implementing preventative measures and lifestyle modifications to mitigate insulin resistance and its associated health risks.

CAUSES AND SYMPTOMS

Insulin resistance is a multifaceted condition influenced by various factors, and its onset is often insidious. Understanding both the causes and symptoms is crucial for early detection and effective management.

Causes:

1. **Genetic Predisposition:**

Inherited factors can contribute to an individual's susceptibility to insulin resistance.

2. **Lifestyle Choices:**

- **Poor Diet:** Diets high in processed foods, sugars, and saturated fats contribute to obesity and insulin resistance.

- **Physical Inactivity:** Sedentary lifestyles reduce insulin sensitivity, promoting the development of resistance.

3. **Obesity:**

Excess body fat, particularly around the abdomen, is strongly correlated with insulin resistance.

4. **Hormonal Imbalances:**

Conditions such as polycystic ovary syndrome (PCOS) and disruptions in other hormones can contribute to insulin resistance.

5. **Inflammation:**

Chronic low-grade inflammation, often linked to obesity and unhealthy diets, interferes with insulin signaling.

6. **Age:**

Aging is associated with changes in metabolism and body composition that can contribute to insulin resistance.

Symptoms:

1. **Increased Hunger:**

Insulin resistance can lead to elevated insulin levels, triggering increased hunger and cravings.

2. **Weight Gain:**

Difficulty in maintaining or losing weight, especially around the abdominal area, is a common symptom.

3. **Fatigue:**

Cells are unable to efficiently utilize glucose for energy, leading to persistent fatigue.

4. **High Blood Sugar Levels:**

Insulin resistance results in elevated blood glucose levels, a precursor to type 2 diabetes.

5. **Frequent Urination:**

Increased blood sugar levels can lead to excessive thirst and frequent urination.

6. **Acanthosis Nigricans:**

Darkened, velvety patches of skin, particularly around the neck and armpits, may indicate insulin resistance.

7. **PCOS in Women:**

Irregular menstrual cycles, infertility, and other symptoms may be associated with insulin resistance in women with PCOS.

CHAPTER TWO

Importance of Insulin Sensitivity

Connection to Overall Metabolic Health

The connection between insulin resistance and overall metabolic health is profound, influencing various physiological processes throughout the body. Insulin, a hormone produced by the pancreas, plays a central role in regulating metabolism. When insulin resistance occurs, disrupting the normal responsiveness of cells to insulin, it has far-reaching implications for metabolic health. Here's an exploration of this connection:

1. Glucose Metabolism:

- Insulin resistance directly affects glucose metabolism. Cells, particularly in muscle, liver, and adipose tissue, struggle to take up glucose efficiently. This leads to elevated blood sugar levels, a hallmark of insulin resistance.

2. Energy Homeostasis:

- Insulin is involved in energy homeostasis by facilitating the storage of excess glucose as glycogen in the liver and muscles. Insulin resistance disrupts this process, contributing to metabolic dysregulation and increased fat storage.

3. Lipid Metabolism:

- Insulin resistance is often associated with dyslipidemia, characterized by elevated triglycerides and reduced high-density lipoprotein (HDL) cholesterol. This imbalance in lipid metabolism contributes to atherosclerosis and cardiovascular risk.

4. Inflammation:

- Insulin resistance is linked to chronic low-grade inflammation. Elevated levels of inflammatory markers negatively impact metabolic health and can contribute to the development of conditions like cardiovascular disease.

5. Hormonal Imbalances:

- Insulin resistance can disrupt the balance of other hormones, such as adiponectin and leptin, which play roles in appetite regulation and energy expenditure. These imbalances further contribute to metabolic dysfunction.

6. Pancreatic Function:

- As insulin resistance progresses, the pancreas often compensates by producing more insulin to maintain normal blood sugar levels. Over time, this increased demand can strain pancreatic function, potentially leading to beta-cell dysfunction and a decline in insulin production.

7. Type 2 Diabetes Risk:

- Prolonged insulin resistance is a major risk factor for the development of type 2 diabetes, a condition characterized by chronic hyperglycemia and further metabolic complications.

8. Cardiovascular Health:

- Insulin resistance is closely tied to an increased risk of cardiovascular diseases, including hypertension, atherosclerosis, and coronary artery disease.

Role in Preventing Type 2 Diabetes

Insulin resistance plays a pivotal role in the development of type 2 diabetes, making its understanding and management crucial in preventing the onset of this metabolic disorder.

Here's an exploration of how addressing insulin resistance is key to preventing type 2 diabetes:

1. Primary Precursor to Type 2 Diabetes:

- Insulin resistance is a primary precursor to type 2 diabetes. When cells become less responsive to insulin, glucose uptake is impaired, leading to elevated blood sugar levels.

2. Compensatory Hyperinsulinemia:

- As the body attempts to overcome insulin resistance, the pancreas produces more insulin to maintain normal blood glucose levels. Prolonged compensatory hyperinsulinemia can contribute to beta-cell exhaustion and dysfunction.

3. Progression to Impaired Glucose Tolerance (IGT) and Impaired Fasting Glucose (IFG):

- Insulin resistance often progresses to conditions like impaired glucose tolerance (IGT) and impaired fasting glucose (IFG), intermediate stages between normal glucose metabolism and overt diabetes.

*

4. Glucotoxicity and Lipotoxicity:

- Elevated glucose levels resulting from insulin resistance can lead to glucotoxicity, causing damage to pancreatic beta cells. Additionally, lipotoxicity, an excess of circulating fatty acids, contributes to beta-cell dysfunction.

5. Inflammation and Oxidative Stress:

- Insulin resistance is associated with chronic inflammation and oxidative stress, promoting the development of diabetes. Inflammatory processes contribute to the impairment of insulin signaling pathways.

6. Preventing the Onset of Type 2 Diabetes:

- Addressing insulin resistance through lifestyle modifications, including a balanced diet, regular physical activity, and weight management, is instrumental in preventing the progression of type 2 diabetes.

7. Medication Interventions:

- Certain medications, such as insulin sensitizers and other antidiabetic drugs, can be prescribed to manage insulin resistance and help prevent the progression of diabetes.

8. Education and Early Intervention:

- Public health initiatives that focus on educating individuals about the impact of lifestyle on insulin sensitivity and diabetes risk can encourage early intervention, fostering preventive measures before the onset of full-blown diabetes.

-

9. Monitoring Blood Sugar Levels:

- Regular monitoring of blood sugar levels is crucial for individuals at risk of insulin resistance. Early detection allows for timely intervention and lifestyle adjustments.

10. Holistic Approach to Health:

- Emphasizing a holistic approach to health, including stress management, adequate sleep, and overall well-being, complements lifestyle changes and contributes to preventing type 2 diabetes associated with insulin resistance.

Types of Insulin Resistance

insulin resistance can manifest in various ways, affecting different tissues and organs in the body. Understanding the types of insulin resistance helps elucidate the complexity of this condition.

Here are two primary types:

1. Tissue-Specific Insulin Resistance:

- **Muscle Tissue Insulin Resistance:** Muscle cells are a major target for insulin's action, facilitating glucose uptake for energy. In insulin resistance, muscle cells become less responsive to insulin, leading to impaired glucose uptake. This contributes to elevated blood sugar levels and reduced energy utilization.

- **Liver Tissue Insulin Resistance:** The liver plays a crucial role in regulating blood glucose levels. Insulin normally inhibits glucose production by the liver. In insulin resistance, the liver becomes less sensitive to insulin, leading to increased glucose production (gluconeogenesis), further contributing to hyperglycemia.

2. Systemic (Whole-Body) Insulin Resistance:

- **Adipose Tissue Insulin Resistance:** Adipose tissue, or fat cells, also exhibit insulin resistance. This leads to an impaired ability to store excess energy as fat, resulting in elevated circulating levels of fatty acids and contributing to lipid-related complications.

- **Pancreatic Beta-Cell Insulin Resistance:** Insulin resistance can affect the pancreatic beta cells, which are responsible for producing insulin. Over time, as insulin demand increases due to peripheral insulin resistance, the beta cells may face challenges in maintaining sufficient insulin production. This can lead to beta-cell dysfunction and a decline in insulin secretion, further exacerbating insulin resistance.

Understanding the tissue-specific nature of insulin resistance provides insights into its diverse manifestations. While muscle, liver, adipose tissue, and pancreatic beta cells are commonly affected, the degree of involvement can vary among individuals.

These types of insulin resistance are often interconnected and contribute to a systemic disruption of glucose and lipid metabolism. Additionally, insulin resistance is not an all-or-nothing phenomenon; it exists on a spectrum, with varying degrees of severity. Lifestyle modifications, such as a healthy diet and regular exercise, along with targeted medical interventions, aim to improve insulin sensitivity and mitigate the impact of insulin resistance on overall health.

CHAPTER THREE

Common Misconceptions About Insulin Resistance

Dispelling Myths and Misunderstandings

Dispelling myths and addressing misunderstandings about insulin resistance is crucial for promoting accurate information and fostering better health outcomes. Addressing these myths helps individuals make informed decisions about their health and encourages a comprehensive approach to preventing and managing insulin resistance.

Here are some common myths associated with insulin resistance, along with clarifications:

Myth 1: Insulin Resistance Only Affects People with Diabetes.

Clarification: Insulin resistance can occur in individuals without diabetes. It's a precursor to type 2 diabetes, but it can also be present in those with prediabetes or metabolic syndrome. Early detection and intervention can help prevent the progression of diabetes.

Myth 2: Only Overweight or Obese Individuals Experience Insulin Resistance.

Clarification: While excess weight is a significant risk factor, insulin resistance can affect individuals with a normal body weight. Genetics, sedentary lifestyles, and poor dietary choices contribute to insulin resistance in people with various body compositions.

Myth 3: Insulin Resistance is Irreversible.

Clarification: Insulin resistance is often reversible, especially in its early stages.

Lifestyle modifications such as a balanced diet, regular exercise, and weight management can improve insulin sensitivity. Medications may also be prescribed to assist in managing insulin resistance.

Myth 4: Insulin Resistance is Solely Caused by Sugar Consumption.

Clarification: While excessive sugar intake contributes to insulin resistance, it's just one factor. Diets high in saturated fats, processed foods, and lack of physical activity also play significant roles. A holistic approach to nutrition and lifestyle is essential for preventing and managing insulin resistance.

Myth 5: Only Older Adults Experience Insulin Resistance.

Clarification: Insulin resistance can occur at any age. However, the risk tends to increase with age due to factors like changes in body composition and metabolic rate. Unhealthy lifestyles can accelerate the onset of insulin resistance in younger individuals.

Myth 6: Insulin Resistance Only Affects Blood Sugar Levels.

Clarification: Insulin resistance has broader effects on metabolism. It influences lipid metabolism, contributes to inflammation, and affects hormonal balance. Addressing insulin resistance is essential not only for blood sugar control but also for overall metabolic health.

Myth 7: All Carbohydrates Are Bad for Insulin Resistance.

Clarification: It's not about avoiding all carbohydrates but choosing the right ones. Whole grains, fruits, and vegetables are part of a healthy diet. The focus should be on complex carbohydrates with high fiber content, which have a smaller impact on blood sugar levels.

Myth 8: If You Have Insulin Resistance, You'll Always Develop Diabetes.

Clarification: While insulin resistance increases the risk of diabetes, it doesn't guarantee its development. Early detection and proactive lifestyle changes can significantly reduce the risk and even reverse insulin resistance in some cases.

Clarifying the Relationship Between Insulin and Weight Gain

While insulin plays a role in fat storage, it is not the sole determinant of weight gain. The interplay of various factors, including diet, physical activity, and individual metabolic responses, contributes to overall weight management and health. A balanced approach that considers the quality of calories, portion sizes, and lifestyle factors is essential for maintaining a healthy weight and preventing insulin-related issues.

The relationship between insulin and weight gain is often a topic of confusion and misinformation. It's essential to clarify how insulin functions in the body and its role in weight regulation:

1. Insulin's Primary Function:

- **Clarification:** Insulin is a hormone produced by the pancreas that plays a central role in regulating blood sugar levels. Its primary function is to facilitate the uptake of glucose by cells for energy. Insulin also promotes the storage of excess glucose as glycogen in the liver and muscles.

2. Insulin and Fat Storage:

- **Clarification:** While insulin facilitates the storage of glucose as glycogen, it also promotes the storage of excess energy in the form of fat. This is a natural and essential process for energy balance. However, issues arise when there is chronic overconsumption of calories, particularly from unhealthy sources.

3. Insulin and Carbohydrate Metabolism:

- **Clarification:** Insulin is released in response to elevated blood sugar levels, typically after consuming carbohydrates. It helps cells take up glucose, preventing excessive sugar in the bloodstream. However, insulin also influences fat metabolism by promoting the storage of fatty acids in adipose tissue.

4. Insulin Resistance and Weight Gain:

- **Clarification:** Insulin resistance, a condition where cells become less responsive to insulin, can contribute to weight gain. As cells resist the actions of insulin, blood sugar levels rise, leading to increased insulin production. This elevated insulin can promote fat storage and inhibit the breakdown of stored fat, contributing to weight gain, especially around the abdominal area.

5. Caloric Balance Matters:

- **Clarification:** Weight gain ultimately depends on the balance between calories consumed and calories expended. While insulin influences fat storage, the overall caloric balance remains a fundamental factor in weight management. Consuming more calories than the body needs, regardless of insulin levels, can lead to weight gain.

6. Type of Calories Matters:

- **Clarification:** The quality of calories matters for overall health. Diets rich in processed foods, sugary beverages, and unhealthy fats can contribute to insulin resistance and weight gain. Choosing nutrient-dense foods, maintaining a balanced diet, and controlling portion sizes are crucial for weight management.

7. Physical Activity and Insulin Sensitivity:

- **Clarification:** Regular physical activity enhances insulin sensitivity. Exercise helps the body use glucose for energy more efficiently and can contribute to weight management.

8. Individual Variability:

- **Clarification:** Individual responses to insulin and dietary factors vary. Some people may be more prone to insulin resistance, while others may have a higher tolerance for certain foods. Personalized approaches to diet and lifestyle are important for optimal health.

CHAPTER FOUR

TREATMENT AND DIAGNOSIS

Diagnosis of Insulin Resistance:

1. Fasting Insulin Test:

- **Procedure:** A blood sample is taken after an overnight fast to measure insulin levels.

- **Interpretation:** Elevated fasting insulin levels may indicate insulin resistance.

2. Oral Glucose Tolerance Test (OGTT):

- **Procedure:** After fasting, the individual drinks a glucose solution, and blood sugar levels are monitored over several hours.

- **Interpretation:** Elevated glucose levels during and after the test may suggest insulin resistance.

3. Hemoglobin A1c (HbA1c) Test:

- **Procedure:** Measures the percentage of hemoglobin with attached glucose molecules, reflecting average blood sugar levels over time.

- **Interpretation:** Higher HbA1c levels may indicate poor glucose control and insulin resistance.

4. Homeostatic Model Assessment for Insulin Resistance (HOMA-IR):

- **Procedure:** Calculated using fasting glucose and insulin levels.

- **Interpretation:** Higher HOMA-IR values suggest insulin resistance.

5. Hyperinsulinemic Euglycemic Clamp:

- **Procedure:** Involves infusing insulin while maintaining blood glucose levels within a normal range.

- **Interpretation:** Measures the body's response to insulin; lower glucose infusion rates indicate insulin resistance.

Treatment and Management of Insulin Resistance:

1. **Lifestyle Modifications:**

   - **Balanced Diet:** Focus on whole foods, fiber-rich fruits and vegetables, lean proteins, and healthy fats. Limit processed foods, sugars, and refined carbohydrates.

   - **Regular Exercise:** Aim for a combination of aerobic and resistance exercises at least 150 minutes per week.

   - **Weight Management:** Achieve and maintain a healthy weight through a balanced diet and regular physical activity.

2. **Medications:**

- **Insulin Sensitizers:** Metformin is a commonly prescribed medication that improves insulin sensitivity and lowers blood sugar levels.

- **Other Antidiabetic Drugs:** Sulfonylureas, thiazolidinediones, and incretin-based therapies may be prescribed based on individual needs.

3. **Blood Sugar Monitoring:**

- Regular self-monitoring of blood sugar levels helps individuals and healthcare providers assess the effectiveness of interventions and adjust treatment plans.

4. **Hormonal Management:**

- For conditions like polycystic ovary syndrome (PCOS), hormonal treatments such as oral contraceptives may be used to regulate menstrual cycles and manage symptoms related to insulin resistance.

5. **Stress Management:**

- Chronic stress can contribute to insulin resistance. Stress-reducing practices, such as mindfulness, meditation, and yoga, may be beneficial.

6. **Treatment of Underlying Conditions:**

- Managing associated conditions like hypertension and dyslipidemia through lifestyle changes and medications is crucial for comprehensive care.

7. **Regular Check-ups:**

- Scheduled follow-ups with healthcare providers allow for continuous monitoring of metabolic markers and adjustments to treatment plans.

8. **Educational Programs:**

- Educational initiatives, including workshops and materials, can help individuals understand insulin resistance, its causes, and the importance of lifestyle modifications.

9. **Individualized Approach:**

- Treatment plans should be tailored to the individual's specific health profile, preferences, and response to interventions.

CHAPTER FIVE

28-DAY MEAL PLANS FOR INSULIN RESISTANCE DIET

Week 1

Day 1:

- **Breakfast:** Greek yogurt with berries and a sprinkle of flaxseeds.

- **Lunch:** Grilled chicken salad with mixed greens, cherry tomatoes, cucumber, and olive oil dressing.

- **Dinner:** Baked salmon with quinoa and steamed broccoli.

Day 2:

- **Breakfast:** Oatmeal topped with sliced almonds, chia seeds, and a dash of cinnamon.

- **Lunch:** Quinoa bowl with black beans, avocado, salsa, and a side of mixed vegetables.

- **Dinner:** Stir-fried tofu with brown rice and a variety of colorful vegetables.

Day 3:

- **Breakfast:** Whole grain toast with smashed avocado and poached eggs.

- **Lunch:** Lentil soup with a side of roasted sweet potatoes and a green salad.

- **Dinner:** Grilled shrimp with asparagus and quinoa.

Day 4:

- **Breakfast:** Smoothie with spinach, berries, banana, and a scoop of protein powder.

- **Lunch:** Turkey and vegetable wrap with a whole grain tortilla.

- **Dinner:** Baked chicken breast with roasted Brussels sprouts and quinoa.

Day 5:

- **Breakfast:** Cottage cheese with pineapple chunks and a handful of walnuts.

- **Lunch:** Quinoa salad with chickpeas, cherry tomatoes, cucumber, and feta cheese.

- **Dinner:** Beef stir-fry with broccoli, bell peppers, and brown rice.

Day 6:

- **Breakfast:** Scrambled eggs with sautéed spinach and whole grain toast.

- **Lunch:** Lentil and vegetable curry with brown rice.

- **Dinner:** Grilled fish tacos with cabbage slaw and avocado.

Day 7:

- **Breakfast:** Whole grain waffles with Greek yogurt and mixed berries.

- **Lunch:** Turkey and vegetable stir-fry with quinoa.

- **Dinner:** Baked cod with roasted sweet potato wedges and green beans.

Week 2

Day 8:

- **Breakfast:** Whole grain pancakes with fresh fruit (berries or sliced banana) and a dollop of Greek yogurt.

- **Lunch:** Chickpea and vegetable stew with a side of quinoa.

- **Dinner:** Baked chicken thighs with sweet potato wedges and steamed broccoli.

Day 9:

- **Breakfast:** Smoothie bowl with spinach, mango, banana, and a sprinkle of chia seeds.

- **Lunch:** Turkey and vegetable lettuce wraps with a side of cherry tomatoes.

- **Dinner:** Grilled salmon with a quinoa and black bean salad.

Day 10:

- **Breakfast:** Scrambled tofu with sautéed kale and whole grain toast.

- **Lunch:** Lentil and vegetable stir-fry with brown rice.

- **Dinner:** Shrimp and vegetable skewers with a side of roasted Brussels sprouts.

Day 11:

- **Breakfast:** Overnight oats with almond butter, sliced strawberries, and a touch of honey.

- **Lunch:** Quinoa and black bean stuffed bell peppers with a side of mixed greens.

- **Dinner:** Baked cod with lemon-herb quinoa and steamed asparagus.

Day 12:

- **Breakfast:** Whole grain English muffin with smashed avocado and poached eggs.

- **Lunch:** Chicken and vegetable kebabs with a side of quinoa.

- **Dinner:** Lentil soup with a side of whole grain bread and a green salad.

Day 13:

- **Breakfast:** Greek yogurt parfait with granola, mixed berries, and a drizzle of honey.

- **Lunch:** Tuna salad lettuce wraps with cherry tomatoes.

- **Dinner:** Grilled chicken breast with roasted sweet potato and green beans.

Day 14:

- **Breakfast:** Whole grain bagel with smoked salmon, cream cheese, and sliced cucumber.

- **Lunch:** Quinoa and vegetable bowl with a tahini dressing.

- **Dinner:** Stir-fried tofu with broccoli and brown rice.

Week 3

Day 15:

- **Breakfast:** Whole grain toast with avocado and poached eggs, paired with a side of mixed berries.

- **Lunch:** Quinoa salad with roasted vegetables, feta cheese, and a balsamic vinaigrette.

- **Dinner:** Grilled shrimp with a quinoa and black bean bowl, topped with fresh cilantro.

Day 16:

- **Breakfast:** Smoothie with spinach, banana, almond milk, and a scoop of protein powder.

- **Lunch:** Turkey and vegetable stir-fry with broccoli, bell peppers, and brown rice.

- **Dinner:** Baked chicken thighs with sweet potato mash and steamed green beans.

Day 17:

- **Breakfast:** Cottage cheese with sliced peaches and a sprinkle of chopped nuts.

- **Lunch:** Lentil soup with a side of whole grain bread and a green salad.

- **Dinner:** Grilled cod with quinoa pilaf and roasted Brussels sprouts.

Day 18:

- **Breakfast:** Whole grain waffles with Greek yogurt, honey, and a mix of fresh berries.

- **Lunch:** Chickpea and vegetable curry with brown rice.

- **Dinner:** Stir-fried tofu with mixed vegetables and quinoa.

Day 19:

- **Breakfast:** Oatmeal topped with sliced almonds, chia seeds, and a handful of diced mango.

- **Lunch:** Quinoa and black bean stuffed bell peppers with a side of guacamole.

- **Dinner:** Baked salmon with lemon-herb quinoa and steamed asparagus.

Day 20:

- **Breakfast:** Scrambled eggs with sautéed spinach and whole grain toast.

- **Lunch:** Chicken and vegetable kebabs with a side of quinoa.

- **Dinner:** Lentil and vegetable stir-fry with brown rice.

Day 21:

- **Breakfast:** Smoothie bowl with mixed berries, banana, granola, and a dollop of Greek yogurt.

- **Lunch:** Tuna salad lettuce wraps with cherry tomatoes.

- **Dinner:** Grilled chicken breast with roasted sweet potato and green beans.

Week 4

Day 22:

- **Breakfast:** Whole grain pancakes with fresh berries and a dollop of Greek yogurt.

- **Lunch:** Shrimp and vegetable stir-fry with broccoli, bell peppers, and brown rice.

- **Dinner:** Baked chicken thighs with quinoa pilaf and roasted Brussels sprouts.

Day 23:

- **Breakfast:** Scrambled tofu with sautéed kale and whole grain toast.

- **Lunch:** Quinoa bowl with black beans, avocado, salsa, and a side of mixed vegetables.

- **Dinner:** Grilled salmon with a quinoa and black bean salad.

Day 24:

- **Breakfast:** Smoothie with spinach, mango, banana, and a sprinkle of chia seeds.

- **Lunch:** Turkey and vegetable lettuce wraps with a side of cherry tomatoes.

- **Dinner:** Stir-fried tofu with broccoli and brown rice.

Day 25:

- **Breakfast:** Greek yogurt parfait with granola, mixed berries, and a drizzle of honey.

- **Lunch:** Quinoa and vegetable bowl with a tahini dressing.

- **Dinner:** Lentil and vegetable stir-fry with brown rice.

Day 26:

- **Breakfast:** Whole grain English muffin with smashed avocado and poached eggs.

- **Lunch:** Lentil and vegetable curry with brown rice.

- **Dinner:** Grilled shrimp with a quinoa and black bean bowl, topped with fresh cilantro.

Day 27:

- **Breakfast:** Oatmeal topped with sliced almonds, chia seeds, and a handful of diced mango.

- **Lunch:** Chickpea and vegetable stew with a side of quinoa.

- **Dinner:** Baked cod with lemon-herb quinoa and steamed asparagus.

Day 28:

- **Breakfast:** Smoothie bowl with mixed berries, banana, granola, and a dollop of Greek yogurt.

- **Lunch:** Tuna salad lettuce wraps with cherry tomatoes.

- **Dinner:** Grilled chicken breast with roasted sweet potato and green beans.

CHAPTER SIX

INSULIN RESISTANCE BREAKFAST FRIENDLY RECIPE

Greek Yogurt Parfait:

Ingredients:

- Greek yogurt
- Berries (strawberries, blueberries)
- Almonds, sliced
- Chia seeds

Instructions:

1. Layer Greek yogurt with berries in a glass.
2. Top with sliced almonds and chia seeds.

- **Nutritional Information (per serving):** Approximately 250 calories, 15g protein, 20g carbohydrates, 12g fat.

Quinoa Breakfast Bowl:

Ingredients:

- Cooked quinoa
- Mixed berries
- Walnuts, chopped
- Honey

Instructions:

1. Combine quinoa with mixed berries.

2. Top with chopped walnuts and a drizzle of honey.

Nutritional Information (per serving): Approximately 300 calories, 8g protein, 45g carbohydrates, 10g fat.

Vegetable Omelette:

Ingredients:

- Eggs

- Spinach

- Tomatoes, diced

- Bell peppers, sliced

- Feta cheese, crumbled

Instructions:

1. Whisk eggs and pour over sautéed vegetables in a pan.

2. Sprinkle with crumbled feta.

- **Nutritional Information (per serving):** Approximately 220 calories, 15g protein, 8g carbohydrates, 14g fat.

Chia Seed Pudding:

- **Ingredients:**

  - Chia seeds

  - Almond milk

  - Vanilla extract

  - Mixed berries

- **Instructions:**

1. Mix chia seeds with almond milk and vanilla extract. Refrigerate overnight.

2. Top with mixed berries before serving.

- **Nutritional Information (per serving):** Approximately 180 calories, 5g protein, 20g carbohydrates, 9g fat.

5. Sweet Potato Toast with Avocado:

- **Ingredients:**

  - Sweet potato slices

- Avocado, mashed

- Cherry tomatoes, sliced

- Red pepper flakes

- **Instructions:**

1. Toast sweet potato slices.

2. Spread mashed avocado and top with cherry tomatoes. Sprinkle with red pepper flakes.

- **Nutritional Information (per serving):** Approximately 220 calories, 3g protein, 30g carbohydrates, 11g fat.

Blueberry Almond Smoothie:

Ingredients:

- Almond milk

- Blueberries

- Almond butter

- Protein powder

Instructions:

1. Blend almond milk, blueberries, almond butter, and protein powder.

2. Serve chilled.

Nutritional Information (per serving): Approximately 250 calories, 15g protein, 20g carbohydrates, 12g fat.

Whole Grain Waffles with Berries:

Ingredients:

- Whole grain waffle mix

- Greek yogurt

- Mixed berries

- Maple syrup (optional)

Instructions:

1. Prepare waffles according to the package.

2. Top with Greek yogurt and mixed berries. Drizzle with maple syrup if desired.

Nutritional Information (per serving): Approximately 280 calories, 10g protein, 40g carbohydrates, 10g fat.

Avocado and Smoked Salmon Toast:

Ingredients:

- Whole grain toast

- Avocado, sliced

- Smoked salmon

- Lemon juice

Instructions:

1. Spread sliced avocado on whole-grain toast.

2. Top with smoked salmon and a squeeze of lemon juice.

Nutritional Information (per serving): Approximately 300 calories, 15g protein, 25g carbohydrates, 16g fat.

Cottage Cheese and Pineapple Bowl:

Ingredients:

- Cottage cheese

- Pineapple chunks

- Almonds, chopped

- Cinnamon

Instructions:

1. Combine cottage cheese with pineapple chunks.

2. Top with chopped almonds and a sprinkle of cinnamon.

   - **Nutritional Information (per serving):** Approximately 220 calories, 15g protein, 20g carbohydrates, 10g fat.

Egg Muffins with Spinach and Feta:

Ingredients:

- Eggs

- Spinach, chopped

- Feta cheese, crumbled

- Cherry tomatoes, halved

Instructions:

1. Whisk eggs and mix with chopped spinach and crumbled feta.

2. Pour into muffin cups, add halved cherry tomatoes, and bake.

Nutritional Information (per serving): Approximately 180 calories, 15g protein, 5g carbohydrates, 12g fat.

Peanut Butter Banana Smoothie:

Ingredients:

- Almond milk

- Banana

- Peanut butter

- Greek yogurt

Instructions:

1. Blend almond milk, banana, peanut butter, and Greek yogurt.

2. Enjoy the smoothie.

Nutritional Information (per serving): Approximately 280 calories, 15g protein, 25g carbohydrates, 14g fat.

Frittata with Vegetables:

Ingredients:

- Eggs

- Bell peppers, diced

- Zucchini, sliced

- Cherry tomatoes, halved

Instructions:

1. Whisk eggs and pour over sautéed vegetables in a pan.

2. Bake until set and golden brown.

- **Nutritional Information (per serving):** Approximately 200 calories, 14g protein, 10g carbohydrates, 12g fat.

Turkey and Vegetable Breakfast Wrap:

Ingredients:

- Whole grain tortilla

- Turkey slices

- Spinach

- Tomatoes, diced

Instructions:

1. Layer turkey slices, spinach, and diced tomatoes on a whole-grain tortilla.

2. Wrap and enjoy.

Nutritional Information (per serving): Approximately 250 calories, 15g protein, 25g carbohydrates, 10g fat.

Almond Flour Pancakes:

Ingredients:

- Almond flour

- Eggs

- Almond milk

- Berries for topping

Instructions:

1. Mix almond flour, eggs, and almond milk to make pancake batter.

2. Cook on a griddle and top with berries.

Nutritional Information (per serving): Approximately 280 calories, 12g protein, 15g carbohydrates, 20g fat.

Salmon and Cream Cheese Bagel:

Ingredients:

- Whole grain bagel
- Smoked salmon
- Cream cheese
- Red onion, thinly sliced

Instructions:

1. Toast the whole-grain bagel.

2. Spread cream cheese, top with smoked salmon, and garnish with red onion slices.

Nutritional Information (per serving): Approximately 320 calories, 20g protein, 30g carbohydrates, 15g fat.

Pumpkin Spice Overnight Oats:

Ingredients:

- Rolled oats
- Almond milk
- Pumpkin puree
- Maple syrup

Instructions:

1. Mix rolled oats, almond milk, pumpkin puree, and a drizzle of maple syrup. Refrigerate overnight.

2. Top with a sprinkle of cinnamon before serving.

Nutritional Information (per serving): Approximately 250 calories, 8g protein, 35g carbohydrates, 10g fat.

Egg and Spinach Breakfast Wrap:

Ingredients:

- Whole grain wrap

- Eggs scrambled

- Spinach, sautéed

- Salsa

Instructions:

1. Fill a whole grain wrap with scrambled eggs, sautéed spinach, and salsa.

2. Roll and enjoy.

Nutritional Information (per serving): Approximately 230 calories, 15g protein, 20g carbohydrates, 10g fat.

Cinnamon Apple Quinoa Bowl:

Ingredients:

- Cooked quinoa

- Apple diced

- Cinnamon

- Walnuts, chopped

Instructions:

1. Combine cooked quinoa with diced apples.

2. Sprinkle with cinnamon and top with chopped walnuts.

Nutritional Information (per serving): Approximately 280 calories, 6g protein, 40g carbohydrates, 10g fat.

CHAPTER SEVEN

INSULIN RESISTANCE LUNCH FRIENDLY RECIPE

Grilled Chicken Salad with Avocado:

Ingredients:

- Grilled chicken breast
- Mixed greens
- Cherry tomatoes
- Cucumber slices
- Avocado slices
- Olive oil and balsamic vinegar dressing

Instructions:

1. Grill the chicken and slice.

2. Toss mixed greens, cherry tomatoes, cucumber, and avocado.

3. Top with grilled chicken and drizzle with dressing.

Nutritional Information (approx.): 350 calories, 30g protein, 15g carbohydrates, 20g fat.

Quinoa and Black Bean Bowl:

Ingredients:

- Cooked quinoa

- Black beans

- Sautéed bell peppers and onions

- Avocado slices

- Fresh cilantro

Instructions:

1. Mix quinoa, black beans, sautéed vegetables, and top with avocado.

2. Garnish with fresh cilantro.

Nutritional Information (approx.): 320 calories, 15g protein, 40g carbohydrates, 12g fat.

Salmon and Vegetable Stir-Fry:

Ingredients:

- Grilled salmon

- Stir-fried broccoli, bell peppers, and snap peas

- Brown rice

- Soy sauce and ginger dressing

Instructions:

1. Grill salmon and set aside.

2. Stir-fry vegetables and toss with brown rice.

3. Top with grilled salmon and drizzle with soy sauce and ginger dressing.

Nutritional Information (approx.): 380 calories, 25g protein, 30g carbohydrates, 18g fat.

Mediterranean Chickpea Salad:

Ingredients:

- Chickpeas
- Cherry tomatoes
- Cucumber, diced
- Kalamata olives
- Feta cheese
- Olive oil and lemon dressing

Instructions:

1. Combine chickpeas, tomatoes, cucumber, olives, and feta.

2. Drizzle with olive oil and lemon dressing.

Nutritional Information (approx.): 290 calories, 12g protein, 30g carbohydrates, 15g fat.

Turkey and Quinoa Stuffed Peppers:

Ingredients:

- Lean ground turkey

- Cooked quinoa

- Bell peppers, halved

- Tomato sauce

- Italian seasoning

Instructions:

1. Cook turkey, mix with quinoa and season with Italian seasoning.

2. Fill bell peppers with the turkey-quinoa mixture.

3. Bake until peppers are tender, and top with tomato sauce.

Nutritional Information (approx.): 310 calories, 25g protein, 30g carbohydrates, 12g fat.

Vegetarian Lentil Soup:

Ingredients:

- Lentils
- Carrots, celery, and onions
- Vegetable broth
- Crushed tomatoes

- Spinach

Instructions:

1. Sauté vegetables, add lentils, broth, and crushed tomatoes.

2. Simmer until lentils are cooked, and stir in spinach.

Nutritional Information (approx.): 250 calories, 15g protein, 40g carbohydrates, 5g fat.

Chicken and Vegetable Quinoa Bowl:

Ingredients:

- Grilled chicken

- Quinoa

- Steamed broccoli, carrots, and snow peas

- Teriyaki sauce

Instructions:

1. Grill chicken and cook quinoa.

2. Assemble the bowl with quinoa, vegetables, and sliced chicken.

3. Drizzle with teriyaki sauce.

Nutritional Information (approx.): 340 calories, 25g protein, 35g carbohydrates, 12g fat.

Shrimp and Avocado Wrap:

Ingredients:

- Grilled shrimp

- Whole grain wrap

- Avocado slices

- Shredded lettuce

- Greek yogurt sauce

Instructions:

1. Fill the wrap with grilled shrimp, avocado, lettuce, and drizzle with Greek yogurt sauce.

Nutritional Information (approx.): 290 calories, 20g protein, 30g carbohydrates, 10g fat.

Roasted Vegetable and Hummus Wrap:

Ingredients:

- Roasted vegetables (zucchini, bell peppers, eggplant)
- Whole grain wrap
- Hummus
- Fresh spinach

Instructions:

1. Fill the wrap with roasted vegetables, spread with hummus, and add fresh spinach.

Nutritional Information (approx.): 280 calories, 10g protein, 35g carbohydrates, 12g fat.

Caprese Chicken Salad:

Ingredients:

- Grilled chicken breast
- Tomatoes, sliced
- Fresh mozzarella, sliced
- Basil leaves
- Balsamic glaze

Instructions:

1. Arrange grilled chicken, tomatoes, and mozzarella on a plate.

2. Garnish with basil leaves and drizzle with balsamic glaze.

- **Nutritional Information (approx.):** 320 calories, 30g protein, 10g carbohydrates, 18g fat.

Tuna and Chickpea Salad:

Ingredients:

- Canned tuna, drained

- Chickpeas

- Cherry tomatoes, halved

- Red onion, diced

- Olive oil and lemon dressing

Instructions:

1. Mix tuna, chickpeas, tomatoes, and red onion.

2. Drizzle with olive oil and lemon dressing.

Nutritional Information (approx.): 280 calories, 25g protein, 20g carbohydrates, 12g fat.

Spinach and Feta Stuffed Chicken Breast:

Ingredients:

- Chicken breast

- Fresh spinach

- Feta cheese

- Garlic powder and black pepper

Instructions:

1. Butterfly chicken breast, stuffed with spinach and feta.

2. Season with garlic powder and black pepper, bake until cooked.

Nutritional Information (approx.): 290 calories, 30g protein, 5g carbohydrates, 15g fat.

Sweet Potato and Chickpea Buddha Bowl:

Ingredients:

- Roasted sweet potato cubes

- Chickpeas, roasted

- Quinoa

- Sliced avocado

- Tahini dressing

Instructions:

1. Assemble bowl with sweet potatoes, chickpeas, quinoa, and avocado.

2. Drizzle with tahini dressing.

Nutritional Information (approx.): 350 calories, 15g protein, 45g carbohydrates, 15g fat.

Eggplant and Tomato Lentil Salad:

Ingredients:

- Lentils, cooked

- Eggplant, grilled and diced

- Cherry tomatoes, halved

- Red wine vinegar dressing

Instructions:

1. Combine lentils, grilled eggplant, and tomatoes.

2. Drizzle with red wine vinegar dressing.

- **Nutritional Information (approx.):** 260 calories, 15g protein, 40g carbohydrates, 8g fat.

Turkey and Vegetable Stir-Fry:

Ingredients:

- Lean ground turkey

- Stir-fried broccoli, bell peppers, and snap peas

- Brown rice

- Soy sauce and ginger dressing

Instructions:

1. Cook turkey and set aside.

2. Stir-fry vegetables, toss with brown rice and add cooked turkey.

3. Drizzle with soy sauce and ginger dressing.

Nutritional Information (approx.): 320 calories, 25g protein, 30g carbohydrates, 12g fat.

Greek Chicken Wrap:

Ingredients:

- Grilled chicken strips

- Whole grain wrap

- Tzatziki sauce

- Sliced cucumber and tomatoes

Instructions:

1. Fill the wrap with grilled chicken, cucumber, and tomatoes.

2. Drizzle with tzatziki sauce.

- **Nutritional Information (approx.):** 310 calories, 30g protein, 30g carbohydrates, 12g fat.

Spaghetti Squash Primavera:

Ingredients:

- Roasted spaghetti squash strands

- Sautéed mixed vegetables (zucchini, cherry tomatoes, bell peppers)

- Olive oil and garlic

Instructions:

4. Sauté vegetables in olive oil and garlic, toss with spaghetti squash.

- **Nutritional Information (approx.):** 240 calories, 5g protein, 30g carbohydrates, 12g fat.

Asian-Inspired Turkey Lettuce Wraps:

Ingredients:

- Ground turkey

- Water chestnuts, diced

- Soy sauce and hoisin sauce

- Butter lettuce leaves

Instructions:

1. Cook turkey, add water chestnuts, and season with soy sauce and hoisin sauce.

2. Spoon into lettuce leaves.

- **Nutritional Information (approx.):** 280 calories, 20g protein, 20g carbohydrates, 14g fat.

Cauliflower Fried Rice with Shrimp:

Ingredients:

- Cauliflower rice

- Shrimp, cooked

- Mixed vegetables (peas, carrots, corn)

- Soy sauce and sesame oil

Instructions:

1. Sauté cauliflower rice, add cooked shrimp and mixed vegetables.

2. Drizzle with soy sauce and sesame oil.

- **Nutritional Information (approx.):** 230 calories, 25g protein, 20g carbohydrates, 10g fat.

Tomato Basil Zoodle Salad with Grilled Chicken:

Ingredients:

- Zucchini noodles (zoodles)

- Cherry tomatoes, halved

- Fresh basil leaves

- Grilled chicken breast

- Balsamic vinaigrette dressing

Instructions:

1. Toss zoodles, tomatoes, and basil.

2. Top with grilled chicken and drizzle with balsamic vinaigrette.

Nutritional Information (approx.): 290 calories, 30g protein, 15g carbohydrates, 15g fat.

CHAPTER EIGHT

INSULIN RESISTANCE DINNER FRIENDLY RECIPE

Baked Salmon with Lemon-Herb Quinoa:

Ingredients:

- Salmon fillet

- Quinoa

- Fresh lemon juice

- Mixed herbs (rosemary, thyme)

- Olive oil

Instructions:

1. Season salmon with herbs, and lemon juice, and bake.

2. Cook quinoa separately and serve with baked salmon.

Nutritional Information (approx.): 350 calories, 30g protein, 25g carbohydrates, 15g fat.

Vegetarian Cauliflower and Chickpea Curry:

Ingredients:

- Cauliflower florets
- Chickpeas
- Coconut milk
- Curry spices (turmeric, cumin, coriander)
- Brown rice

Instructions:

1. Sauté cauliflower and chickpeas in curry spices.

2. Add coconut milk, and simmer until vegetables are tender.

3. Serve over brown rice.

- **Nutritional Information (approx.):** 320 calories, 15g protein, 40g carbohydrates, 12g fat.

Grilled Chicken and Vegetable Skewers:

Ingredients:

- Chicken breast, cubed

- Bell peppers, cherry tomatoes, zucchini

- Olive oil and garlic marinade

Instructions:

1. Marinate chicken in olive oil and garlic.

2. Skewer chicken and vegetables, and grill until cooked.

Nutritional Information (approx.): 280 calories, 25g protein, 20g carbohydrates, 12g fat.

Spaghetti Squash Shrimp Scampi:

Ingredients:

- Spaghetti squash

- Shrimp, peeled and deveined

- Garlic, lemon juice, and parsley

- Olive oil

Instructions:

1. Roast spaghetti squash and scrape into strands.

2. Sauté shrimp with garlic, lemon, and parsley in olive oil.

3. Toss with spaghetti squash.

Nutritional Information (approx.): 300 calories, 20g protein, 30g carbohydrates, 12g fat.

Stuffed Bell Peppers with Turkey and Quinoa:

Ingredients:

- Bell peppers, halved

- Ground turkey

- Cooked quinoa

- Tomato sauce

Instructions:

1. Cook turkey, mix with quinoa and tomato sauce.

2. Fill bell peppers and bake until peppers are tender.

- **Nutritional Information (approx.):** 310 calories, 25g protein, 30g carbohydrates, 12g fat.

Baked Cod with Mediterranean Vegetables:

Ingredients:

- Cod fillet
- Cherry tomatoes, olives, artichokes
- Olive oil and lemon
- Quinoa or couscous

Instructions:

1. Place cod on a baking sheet, and surround it with vegetables.

2. Drizzle with olive oil and lemon, and bake until the fish is cooked.

3. Serve over quinoa or couscous.

Nutritional Information (approx.): 340 calories, 25g protein, 30g carbohydrates, 15g fat.

Eggplant and Tomato Lentil Casserole:

Ingredients:

- Lentils, cooked

- Eggplant, sliced

- Tomatoes, sliced

- Feta cheese

Instructions:

1. Layer lentils, eggplant, and tomatoes in a baking dish.

2. Top with feta cheese and bake until vegetables are tender.

- **Nutritional Information (approx.):** 280 calories, 15g protein, 40g carbohydrates, 8g fat.

Grilled Tofu and Vegetable Skewers:

Ingredients:

- Firm tofu, cubed

- Bell peppers, cherry tomatoes, mushrooms

- Balsamic vinegar and olive oil marinade

Instructions:

1. Marinate tofu and vegetables in balsamic vinegar and olive oil.

2. Skewer and grill until tofu is golden and vegetables are tender.

- **Nutritional Information (approx.):** 260 calories, 20g protein, 20g carbohydrates, 12g fat.

Mushroom and Spinach Stuffed Chicken Breast:

Ingredients:

- Chicken breast

- Sautéed mushrooms and spinach

- Garlic powder and black pepper

Instructions:

1. Butterfly chicken breast, stuffed with mushrooms and spinach.

2. Season with garlic powder and black pepper, bake until cooked.

Nutritional Information (approx.): 290 calories, 30g protein, 5g carbohydrates, 15g fat.

Cauliflower Fried Rice with Chicken:

Ingredients:

- Cauliflower rice

- Grilled chicken, diced

- Mixed vegetables (peas, carrots, corn)

- Soy sauce and sesame oil

Instructions:

1. Sauté cauliflower rice, add grilled chicken and mixed vegetables.

2. Drizzle with soy sauce and sesame oil.

Nutritional Information (approx.): 290 calories, 30g protein, 20g carbohydrates, 12g fat.

Sweet Potato and Chickpea Curry:

Ingredients:

- Sweet potatoes, diced

- Chickpeas

- Coconut milk

- Curry spices (turmeric, cumin, coriander)

- Brown rice

Instructions:

1. Sauté sweet potatoes and chickpeas in curry spices.

2. Add coconut milk, and simmer until vegetables are tender.

3. Serve over brown rice.

Nutritional Information (approx.): 330 calories, 15g protein, 40g carbohydrates, 15g fat.

Zucchini Noodles with Pesto Shrimp:

Ingredients:

- Zucchini noodles (zoodles)
- Shrimp, cooked
- Cherry tomatoes, halved
- Pesto sauce

Instructions:

1. Sauté zucchini noodles, add cooked shrimp and cherry tomatoes.

2. Toss with pesto sauce.

- **Nutritional Information (approx.):** 280 calories, 25g protein, 15g carbohydrates, 14g fat.

Lemon Garlic Chicken and Broccoli Stir-Fry:

Ingredients:

- Chicken breast, sliced

- Broccoli florets

- Garlic, minced

- Lemon juice

- Soy sauce

Instructions:

1. Stir-fry chicken until cooked, add broccoli, garlic, lemon juice, and soy sauce.

Nutritional Information (approx.): 300 calories, 25g protein, 20g carbohydrates, 15g fat.

Sesame Ginger Tofu Stir-Fry:

Ingredients:

- Firm tofu, cubed

- Mixed vegetables (bell peppers, broccoli, snap peas)

- Sesame ginger sauce

- Brown rice

Instructions:

1. Sauté tofu and vegetables, toss with sesame ginger sauce.

2. Serve over brown rice.

Nutritional Information (approx.): 280 calories, 20g protein, 30g carbohydrates, 12g fat.

Mediterranean Quinoa Bowl with Grilled Chicken:

Ingredients:

- Quinoa

- Grilled chicken breast

- Cherry tomatoes, cucumber, olives

- Feta cheese

- Greek dressing

Instructions:

1. Cook quinoa, and assemble bowl with grilled chicken and vegetables.

2. Top with feta cheese and drizzle with Greek dressing.

Nutritional Information (approx.): 340 calories, 30g protein, 25g carbohydrates, 15g fat.

Broccoli and Cheddar Stuffed Baked Potatoes:

Ingredients:

- Baked potatoes

- Steamed broccoli

- Cheddar cheese

- Greek yogurt

Instructions:

1. Scoop out the insides of baked potatoes, and mix with steamed broccoli and cheddar cheese.

2. Stuff the mixture back into the potato skins, and bake until the cheese is melted.

3. Serve with a dollop of Greek yogurt.

Nutritional Information (approx.): 320 calories, 15g protein, 40g carbohydrates, 12g fat.

Teriyaki Salmon with Stir-Fried Vegetables:

Ingredients:

- Salmon fillet
- Teriyaki sauce
- Stir-fried vegetables (broccoli, bell peppers, carrots)
- Brown rice

Instructions:

1. Marinate salmon in teriyaki sauce, and bake until cooked.
2. Serve with stir-fried vegetables and brown rice.

Nutritional Information (approx.): 340 calories, 25g protein, 30g carbohydrates, 15g fat.

Chickpea and Spinach Coconut Curry:

Ingredients:

- Chickpeas
- Fresh spinach
- Coconut milk
- Curry spices (turmeric, cumin, coriander)
- Quinoa or brown rice

Instructions:

1. Simmer chickpeas and spinach in coconut milk with curry spices.
2. Serve over quinoa or brown rice.

- **Nutritional Information (approx.):** 330 calories, 15g protein, 40g carbohydrates, 15g fat.

Mango Lime Grilled Chicken Salad:

Ingredients:

- Grilled chicken breast
- Mixed greens
- Mango slices
- Avocado slices
- Lime vinaigrette dressing

Instructions:

1. Grill chicken, slice, and toss with mixed greens, mango, and avocado.
2. Drizzle with lime vinaigrette dressing.

- **Nutritional Information (approx.):** 350 calories, 30g protein, 20g carbohydrates, 18g fat.

CHAPTER NINE

CONCLUSION

In conclusion, embarking on a journey to manage insulin resistance through a carefully curated cookbook and meal plan for beginners is a transformative step towards improved health and well-being. This comprehensive guide not only equips you with delicious and nutritious recipes but also empowers you to make mindful choices that support insulin sensitivity.

By embracing the principles outlined in this cookbook, you're not just creating meals; you're cultivating a lifestyle that promotes overall health. The recipes provided are not only tasty but thoughtfully designed to balance key nutrients, making them an essential tool in managing insulin resistance.

Remember, this cookbook is a starting point for your culinary adventure, and it encourages you to explore the vibrant world of nutrient-dense, insulin-friendly foods. Each meal is an opportunity to nourish your body, stabilize blood sugar levels, and embark on a path to sustainable well-being.

As you embark on this culinary journey, embrace the joy of experimenting with flavors, textures, and ingredients that support insulin sensitivity. Cultivate an understanding of how food interacts with your body, and savor the positive impact on your overall health.

Ultimately, this insulin resistance cookbook and meal plan for beginners serves as a roadmap toward a healthier lifestyle. It's not just about what you eat; it's about fostering a positive relationship with food and empowering yourself to take charge of your well-being. May these recipes inspire you to make informed choices, enjoy your culinary experiences, and embark on a delicious and fulfilling journey toward a healthier, more balanced life.